Emergency Jobs
ER Doctors

by Julie Murray

Dash!
LEVELED READERS
2
An Imprint of Abdo Zoom • abdobooks.com

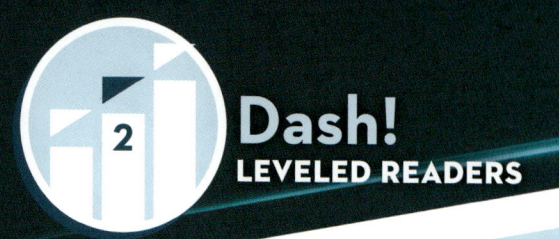

Dash!
LEVELED READERS

Level 1 – Beginning
Short and simple sentences with familiar words or patterns for children who are beginning to understand how letters and sounds go together.

Level 2 – Emerging
Longer words and sentences with more complex language patterns for readers who are practicing common words and letter sounds.

Level 3 – Transitional
More developed language and vocabulary for readers who are becoming more independent.

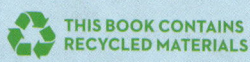
THIS BOOK CONTAINS RECYCLED MATERIALS

abdobooks.com

Published by Abdo Zoom, a division of ABDO, PO Box 398166, Minneapolis, Minnesota 55439. Copyright © 2021 by Abdo Consulting Group, Inc. International copyrights reserved in all countries. No part of this book may be reproduced in any form without written permission from the publisher. Dash!™ is a trademark and logo of Abdo Zoom.

Printed in the United States of America, North Mankato, Minnesota.
102020
012021

Photo Credits: Getty Images, iStock, Shutterstock
Production Contributors: Kenny Abdo, Jennie Forsberg, Grace Hansen, John Hansen
Design Contributors: Dorothy Toth, Neil Klinepier, Laura Graphenteen

Library of Congress Control Number: 2020910994

Publisher's Cataloging in Publication Data

Names: Murray, Julie, author.
Title: ER doctors / by Julie Murray
Description: Minneapolis, Minnesota : Abdo Zoom, 2021 | Series: Emergency jobs | Includes online resources and index.
Identifiers: ISBN 9781098223045 (lib. bdg.) | ISBN 9781098223748 (ebook) | ISBN 9781098224097 (Read-to-Me ebook)
Subjects: LCSH: Physicians--Juvenile literature. | Emergency physicians--Juvenile literature. | Hospitals--Emergency services--Juvenile literature. | Assistance in emergencies--Juvenile literature.
Classification: DDC 363.3481--dc23

Table of Contents

ER Doctors 4

Training. 16

More Facts 22

Glossary 23

Index 24

Online Resources 24

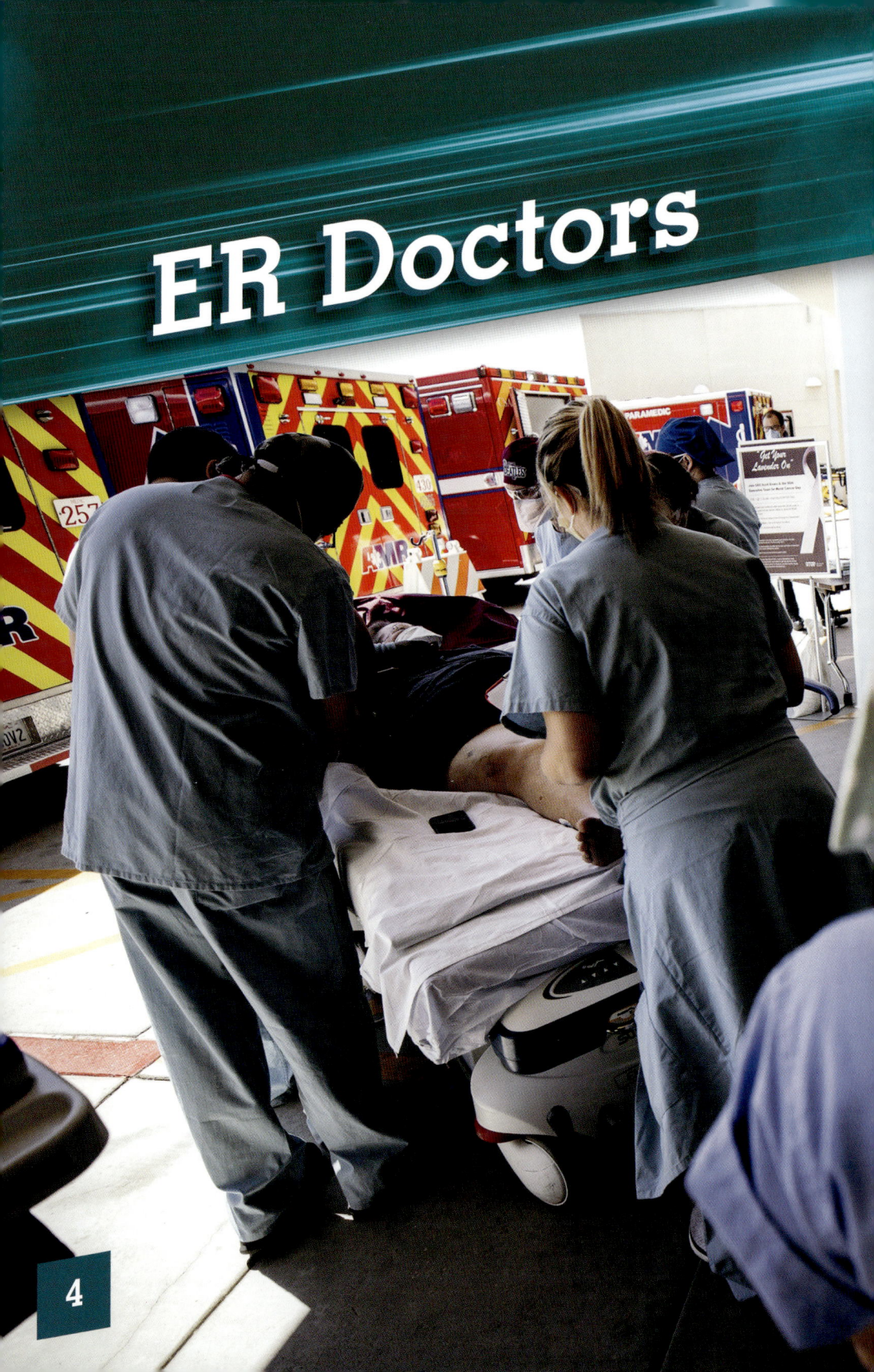

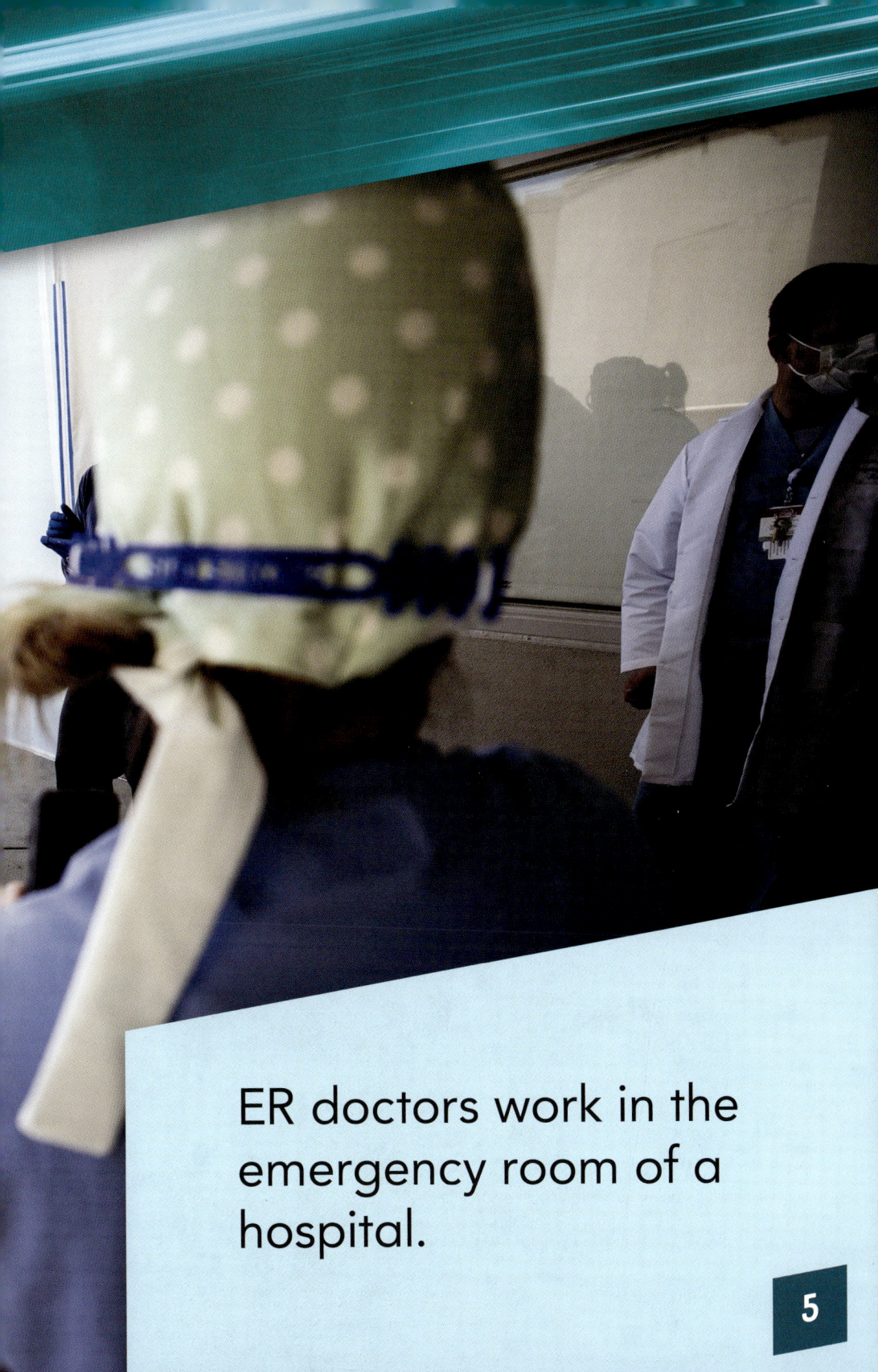

ER doctors work in the emergency room of a hospital.

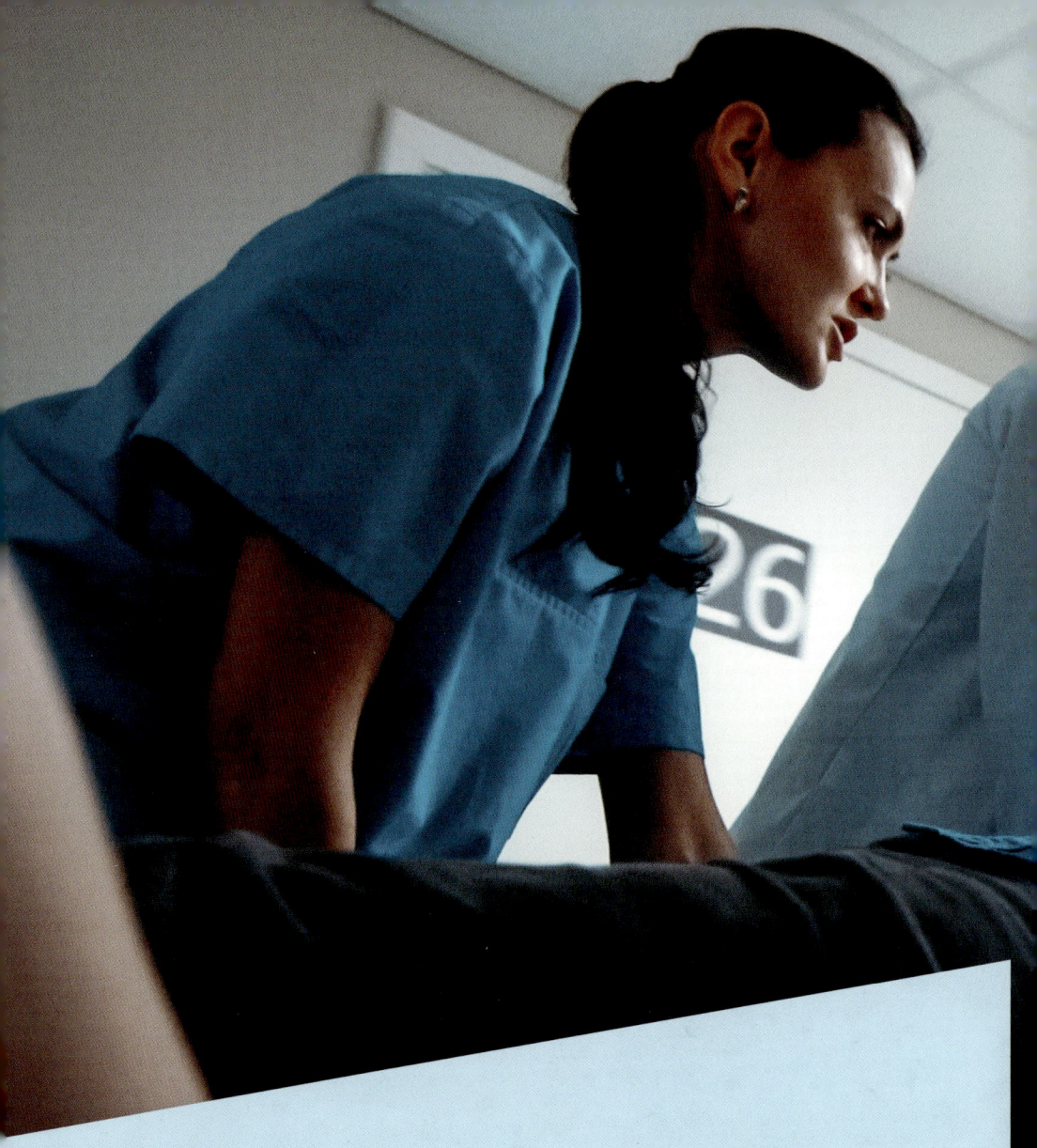

ER doctors treat many issues. They see accident **victims**. They also see people with heart problems.

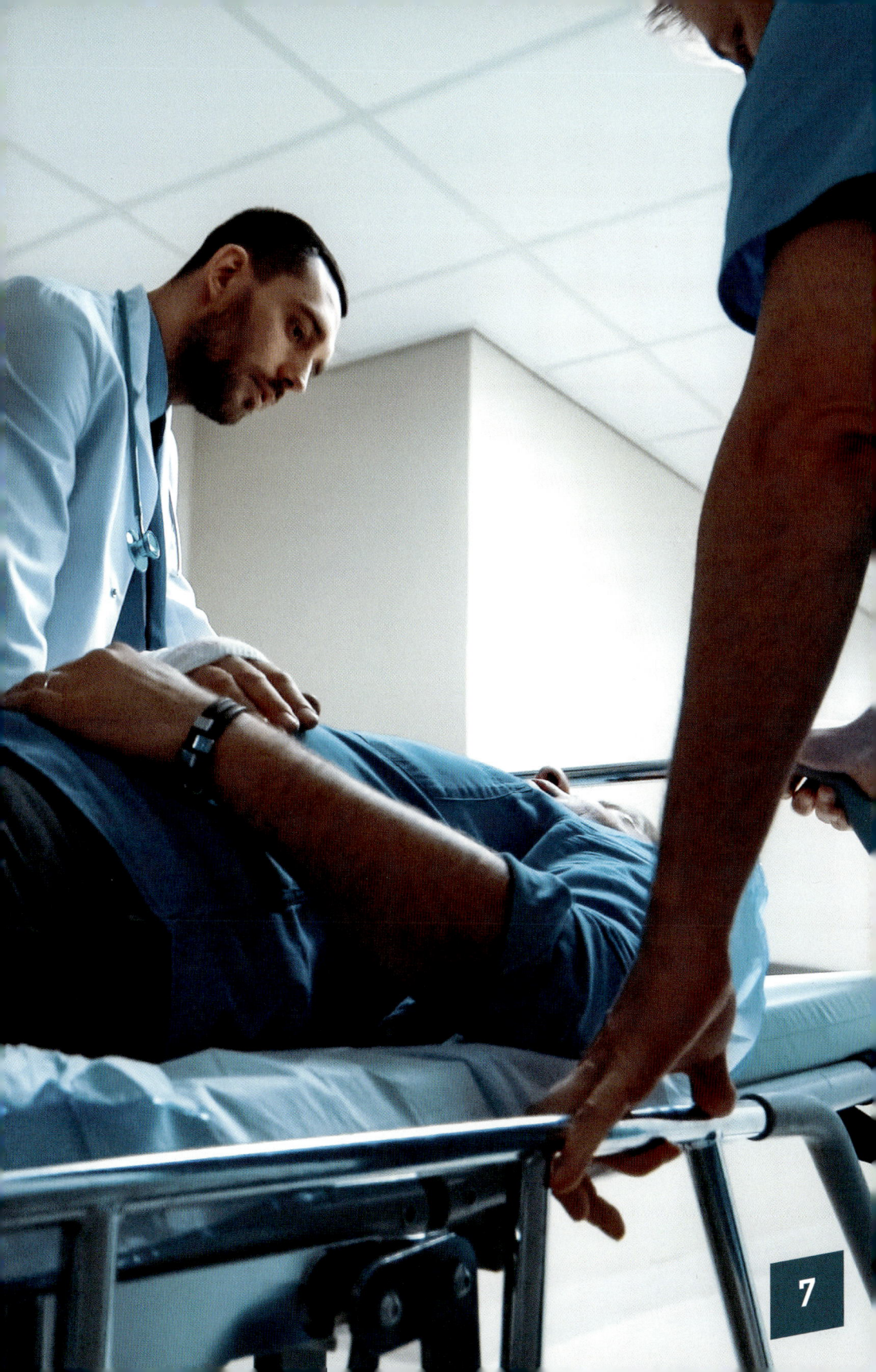

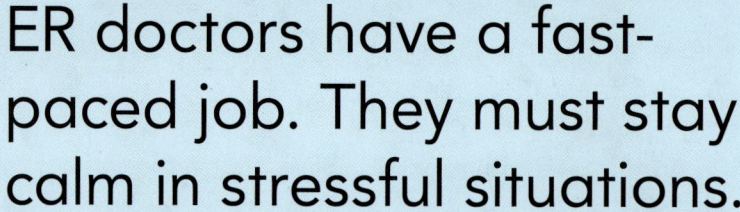

ER doctors have a fast-paced job. They must stay calm in stressful situations.

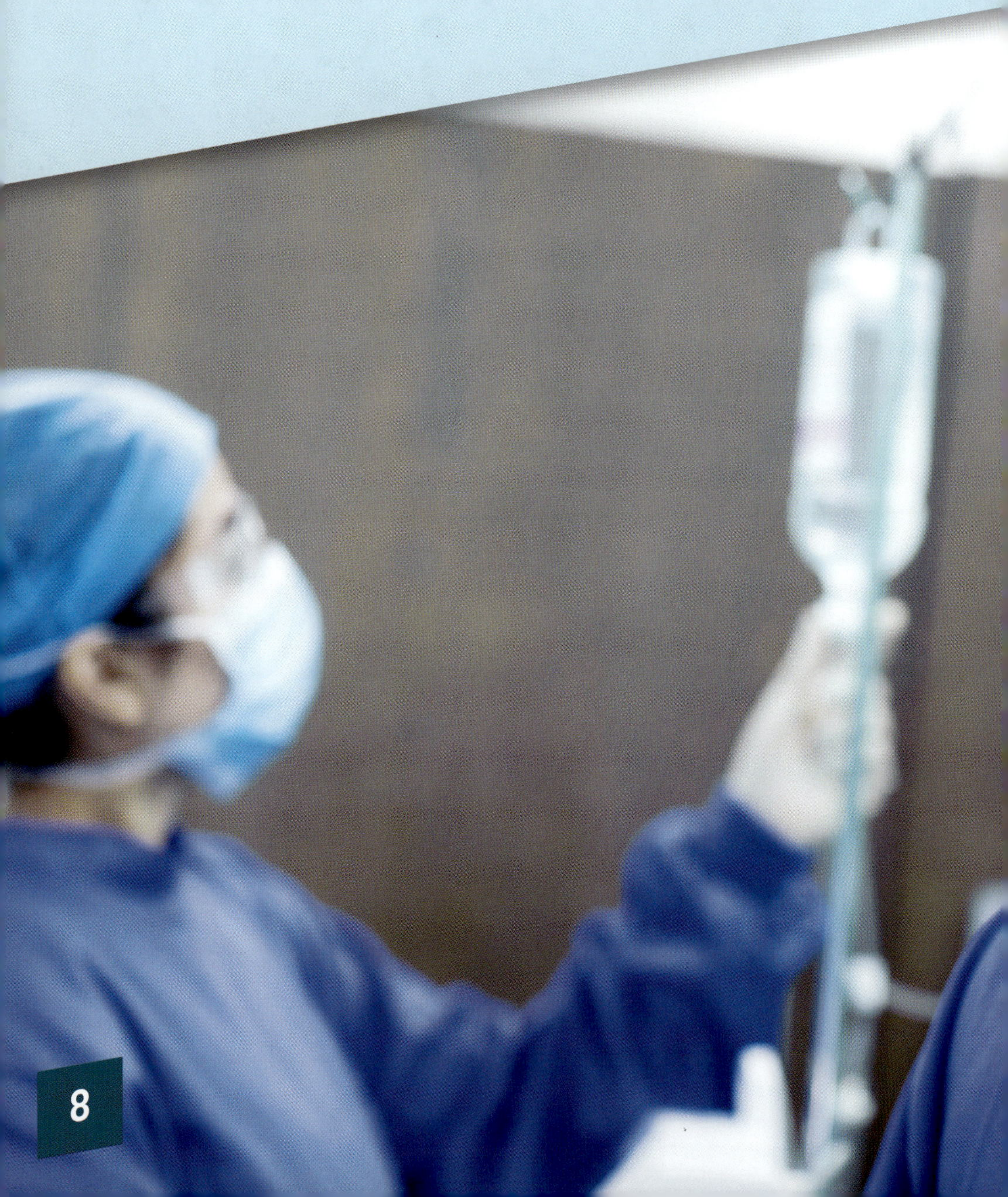

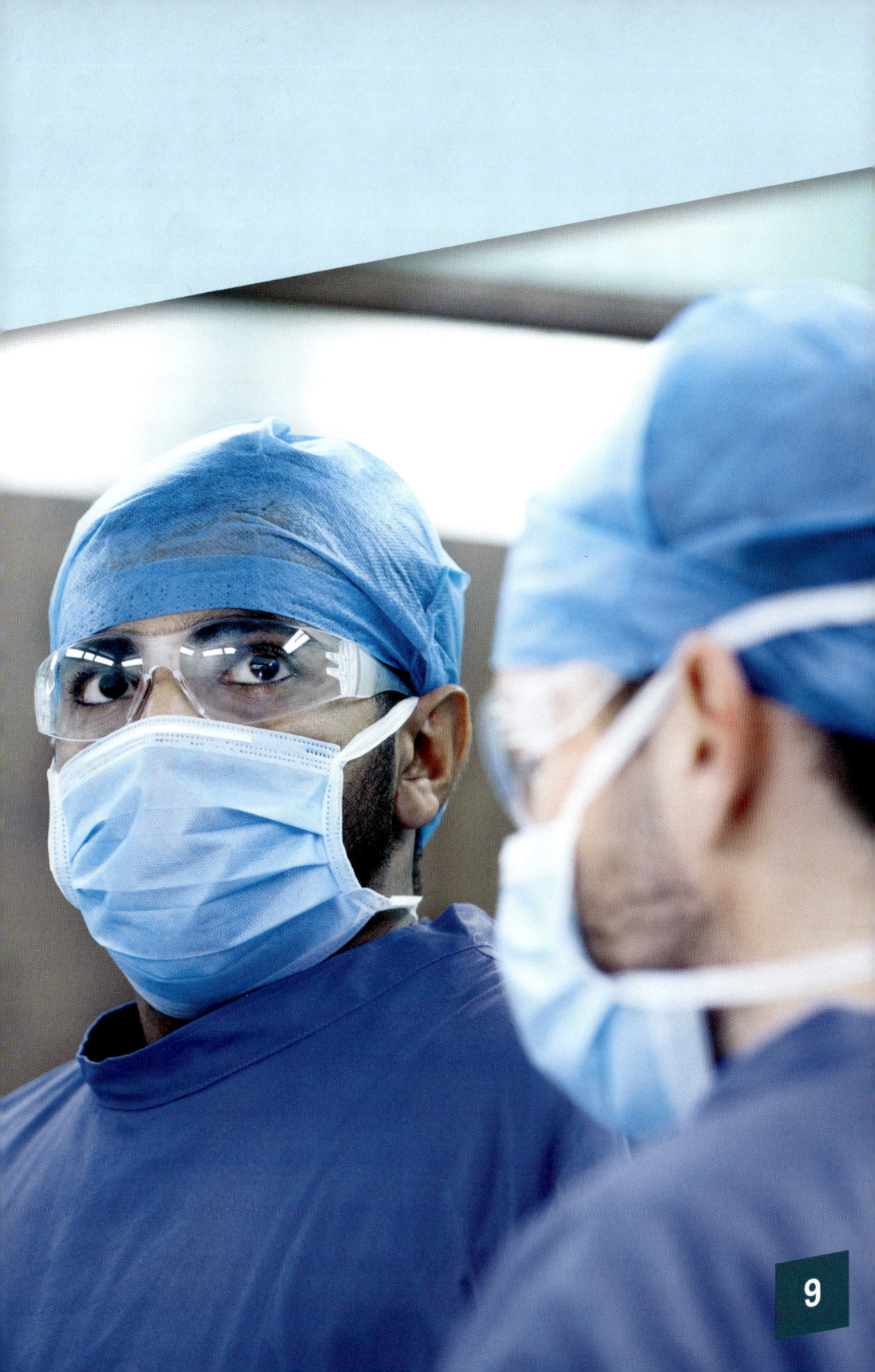

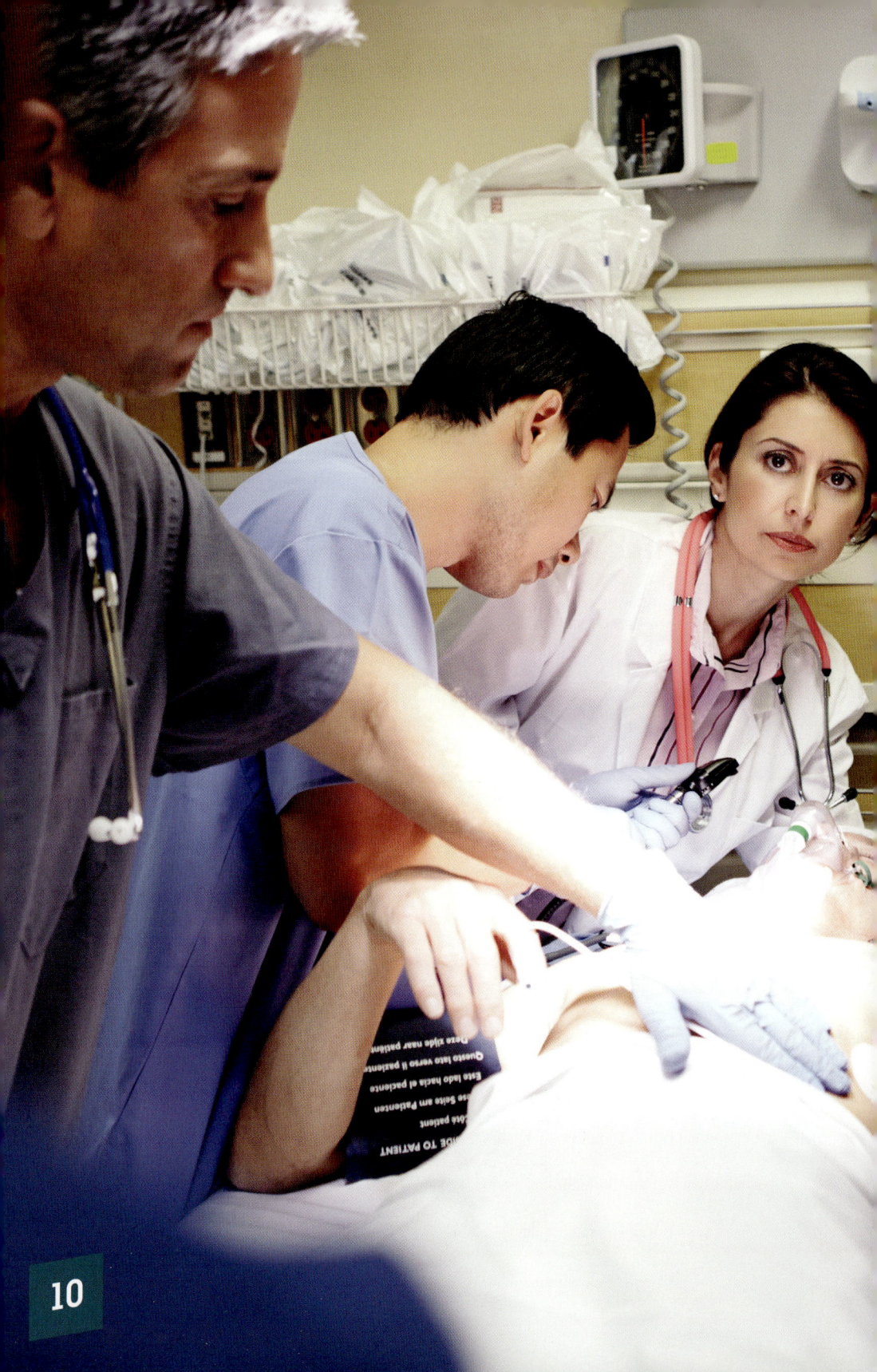

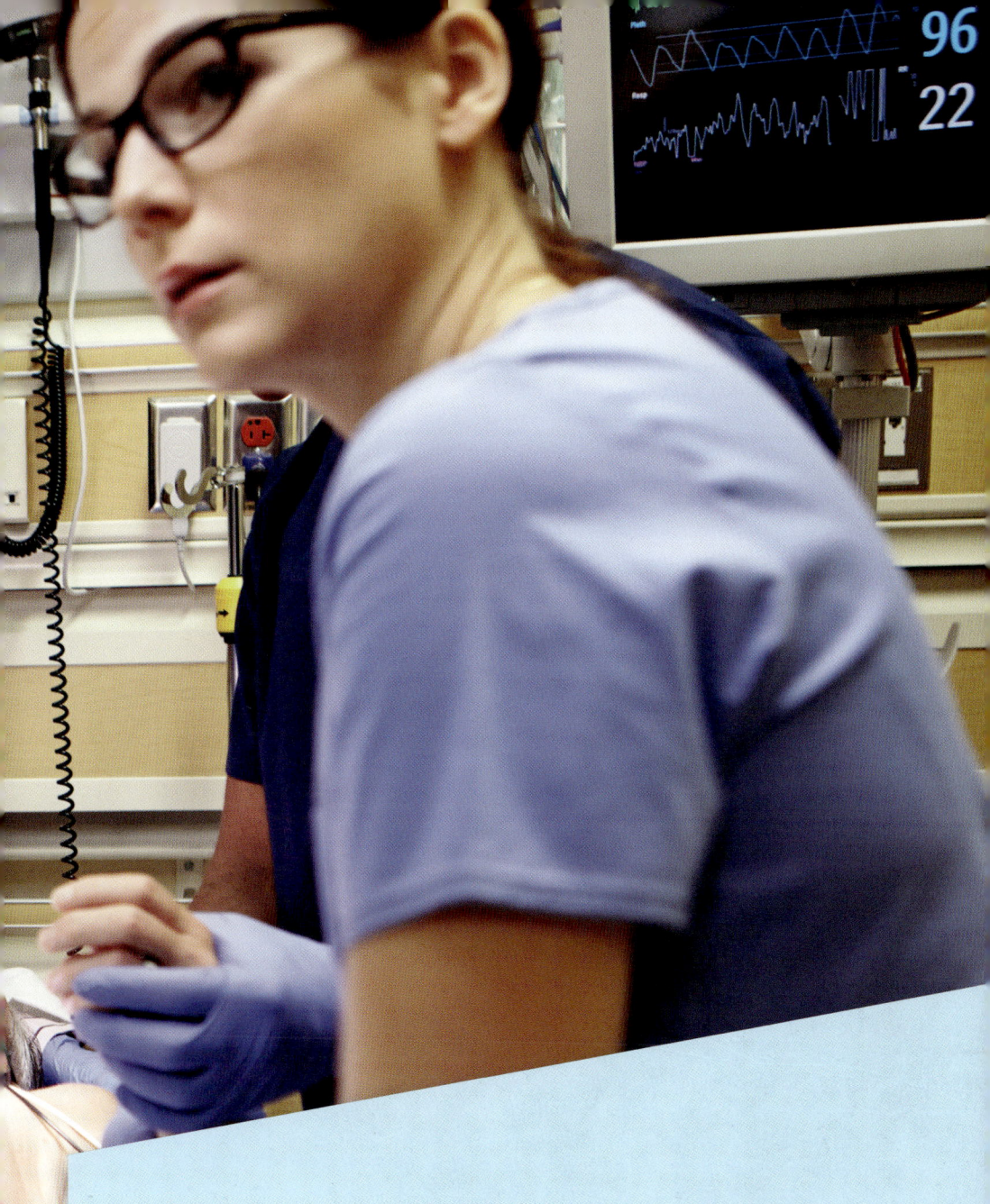

Their first job is to **stabilize** their patients. They order tests to find the problem.

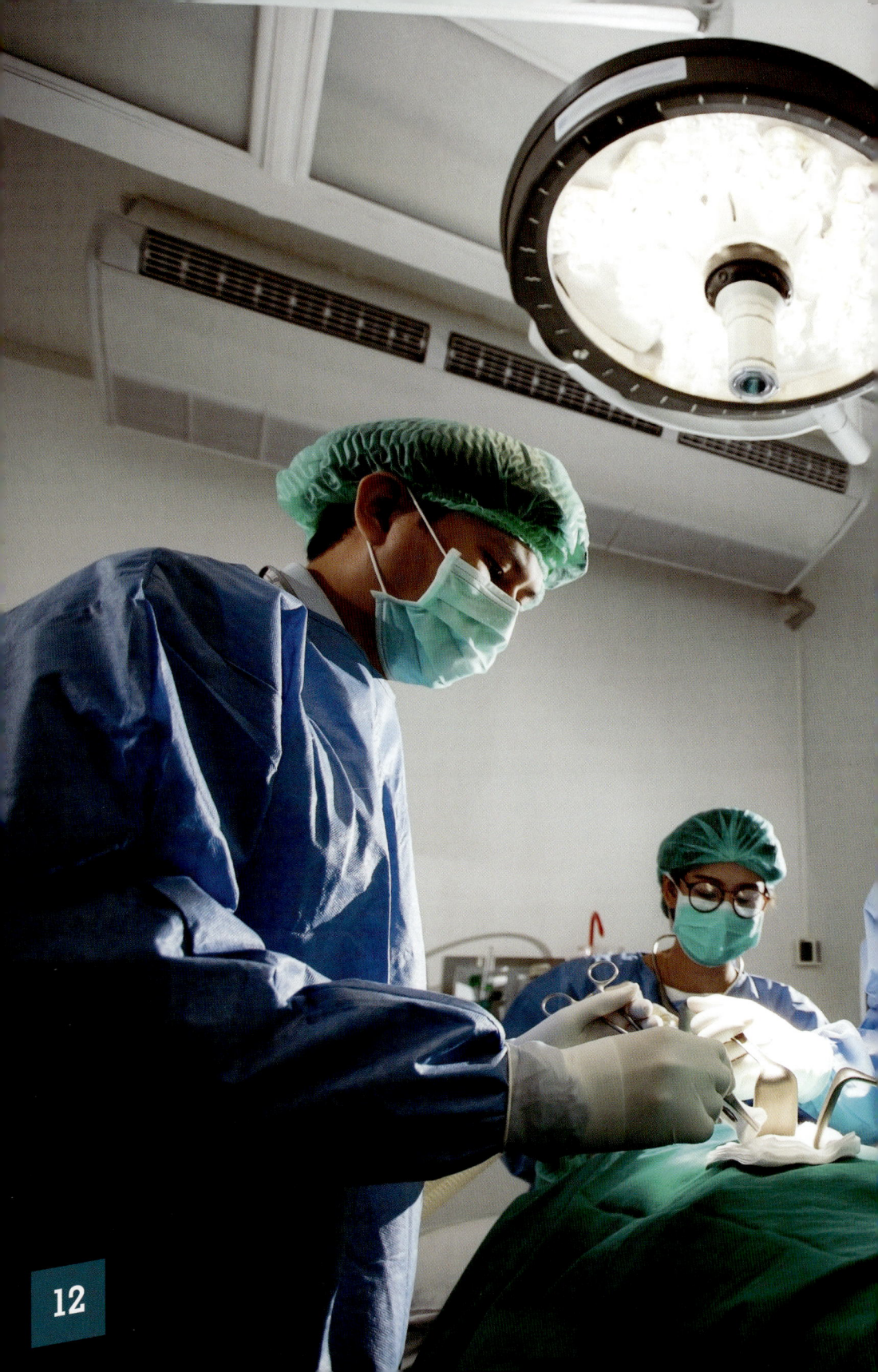

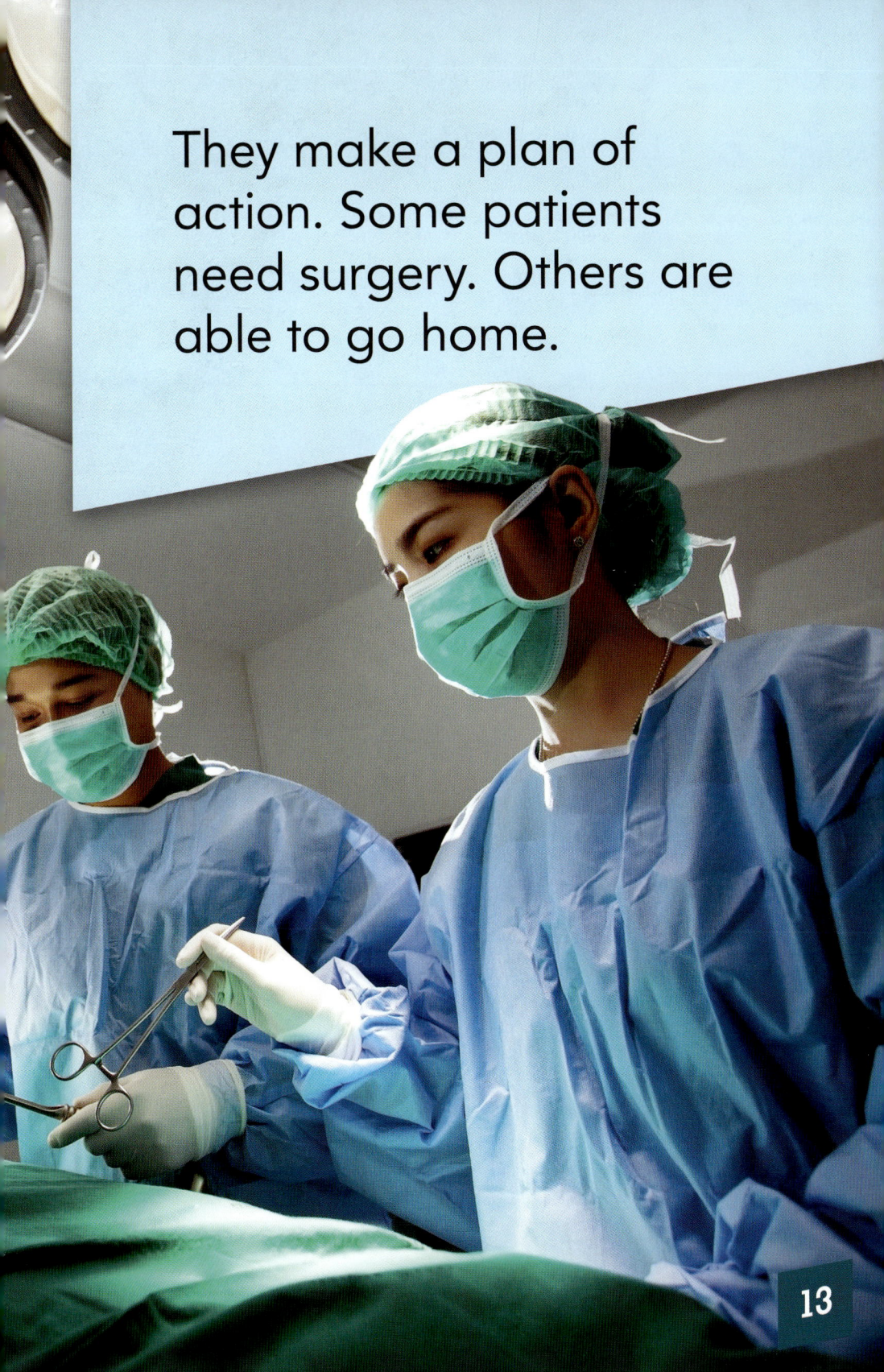

They make a plan of action. Some patients need surgery. Others are able to go home.

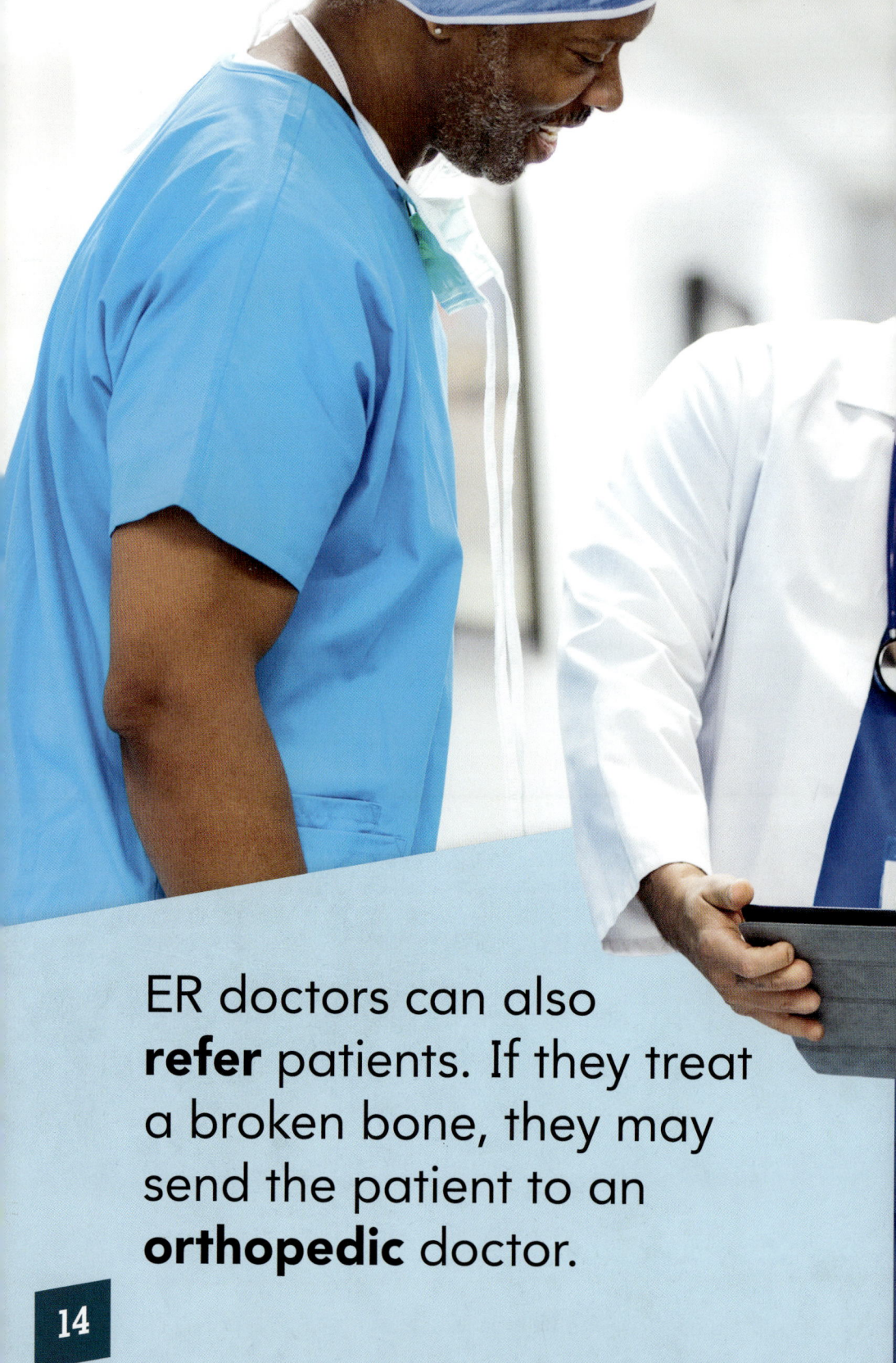

ER doctors can also **refer** patients. If they treat a broken bone, they may send the patient to an **orthopedic** doctor.

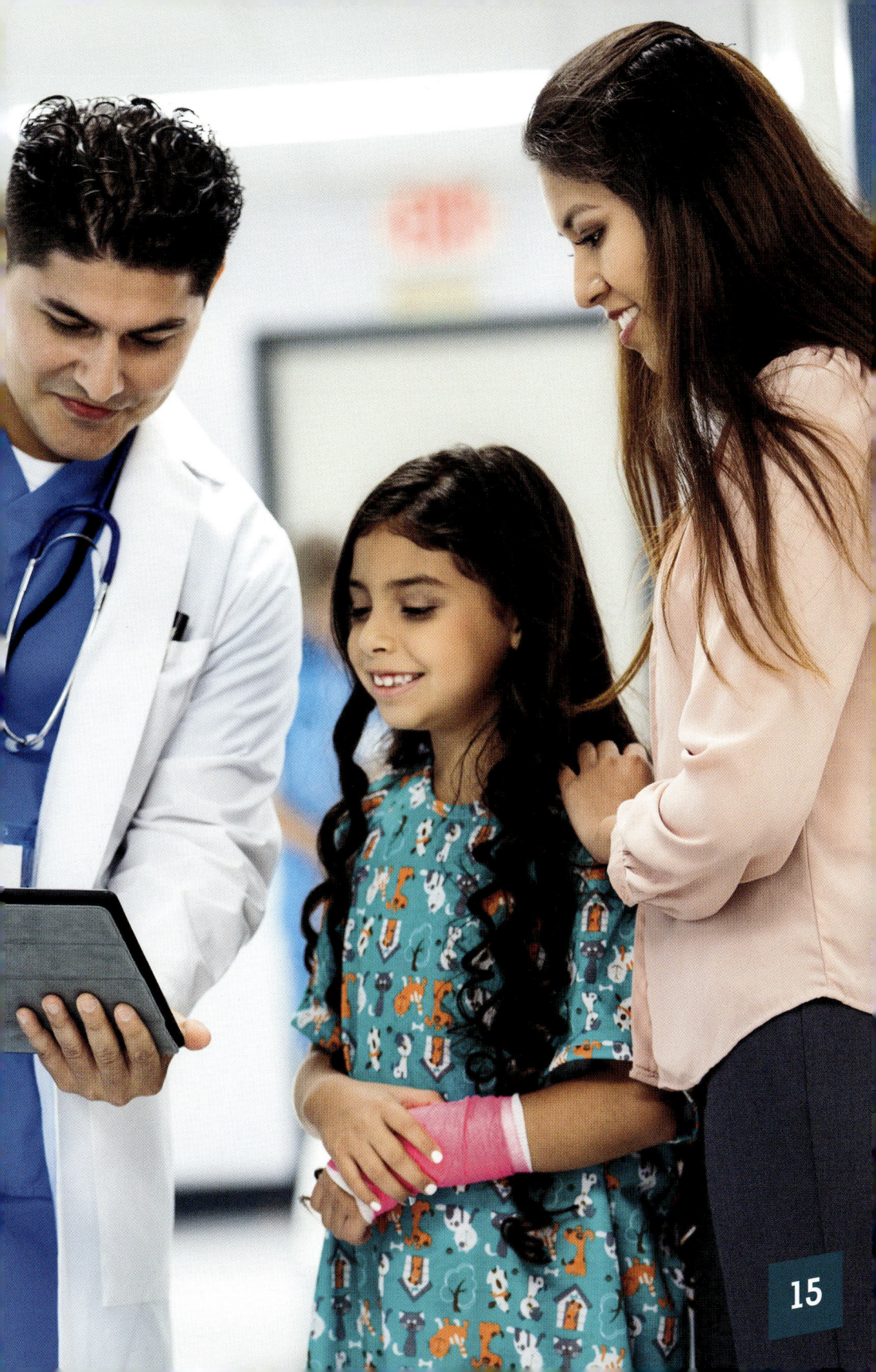

Training

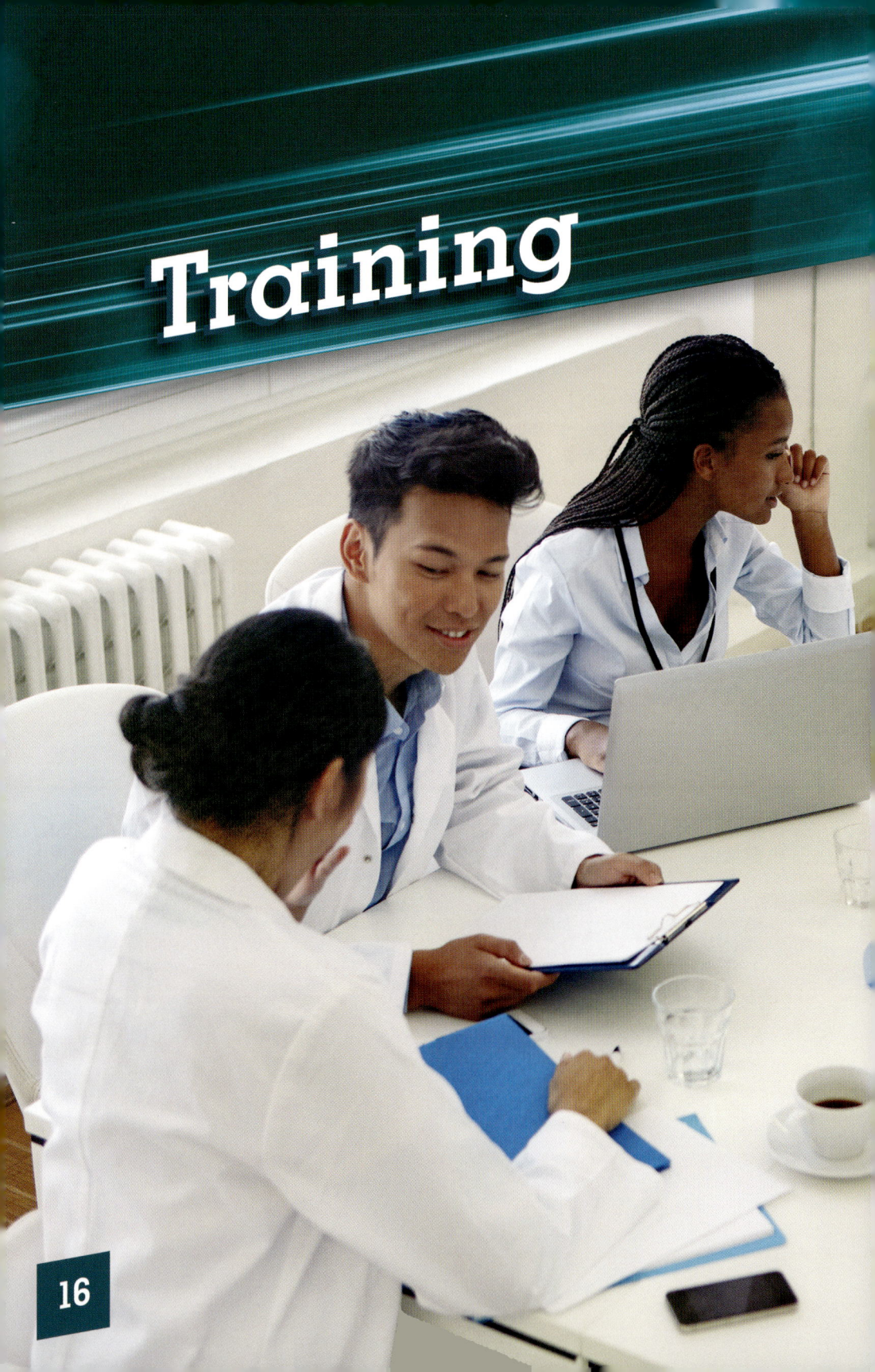

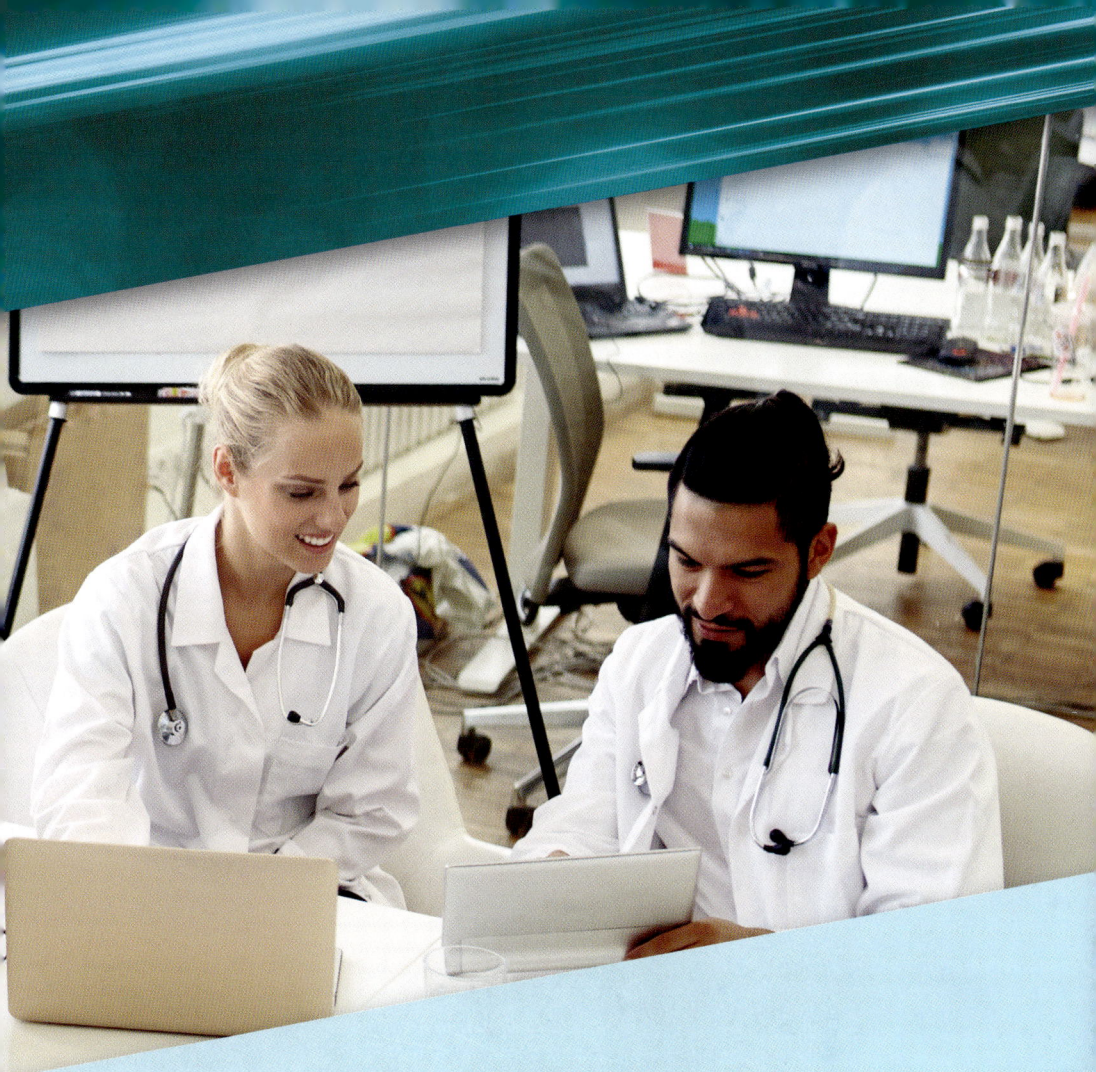

It takes many years of education to be an ER doctor. First, a four-year college degree is needed. Then a student attends four years of medical school.

A **residency** in emergency medicine is also needed. It can last three to four years.

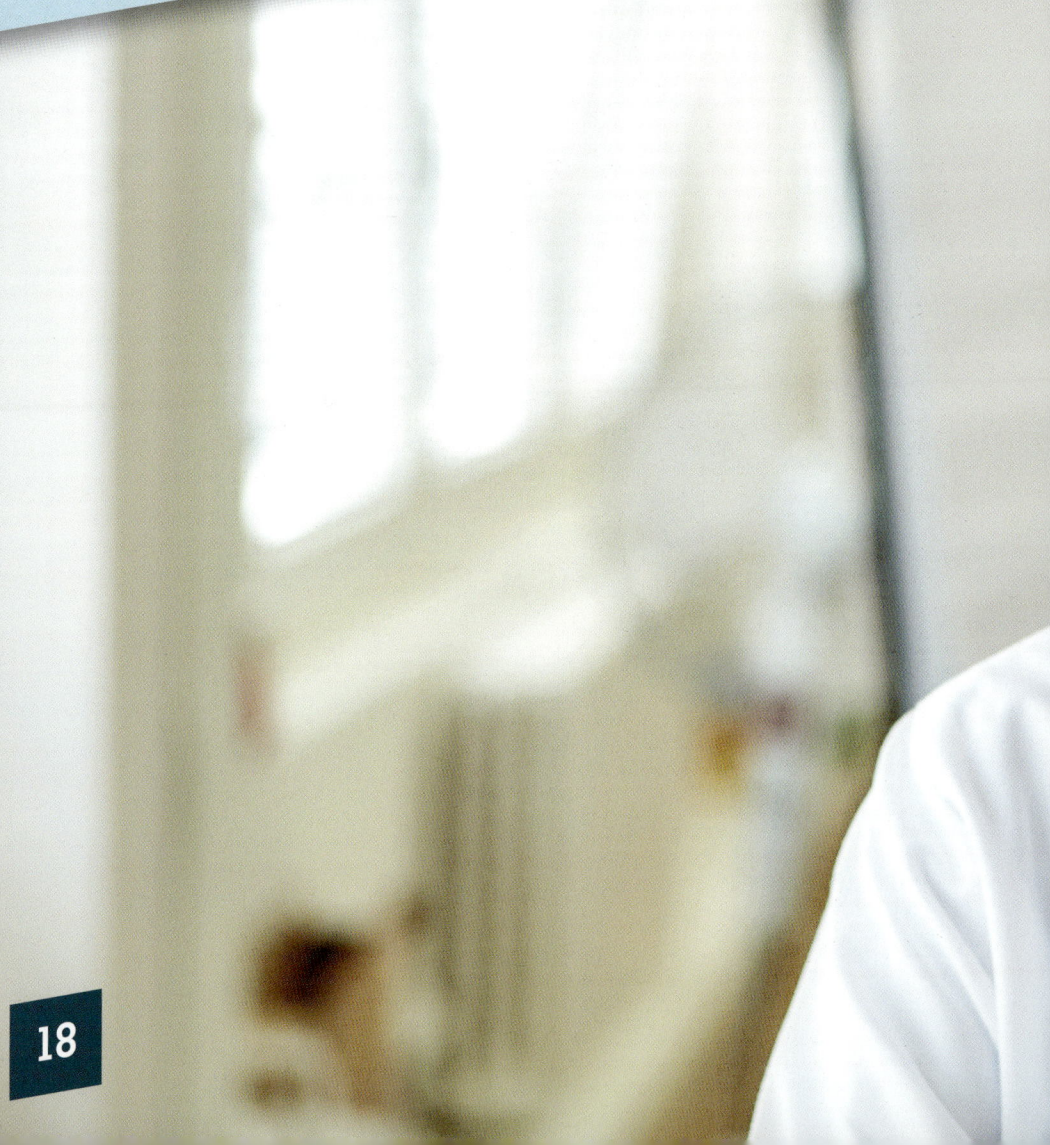

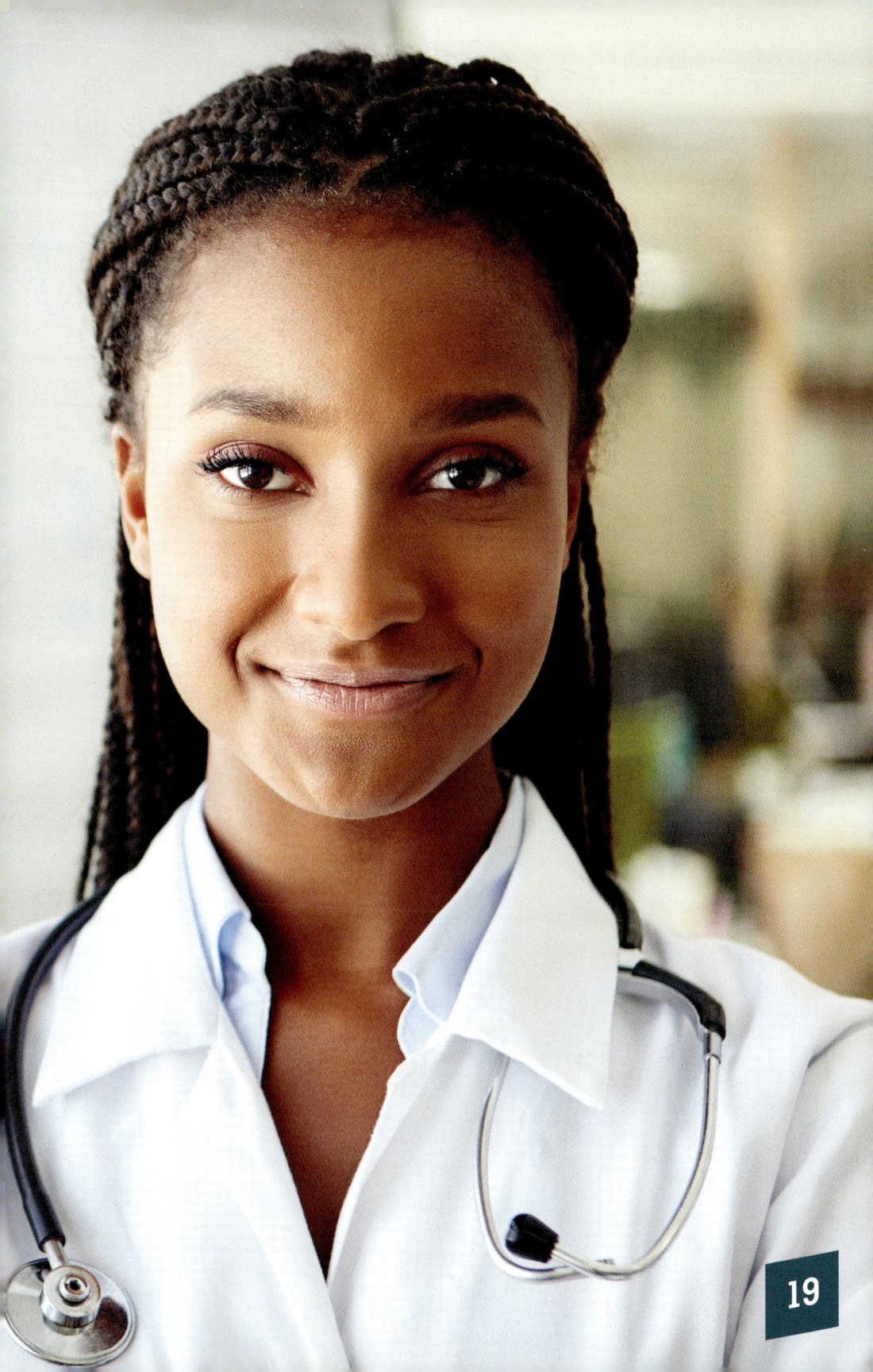

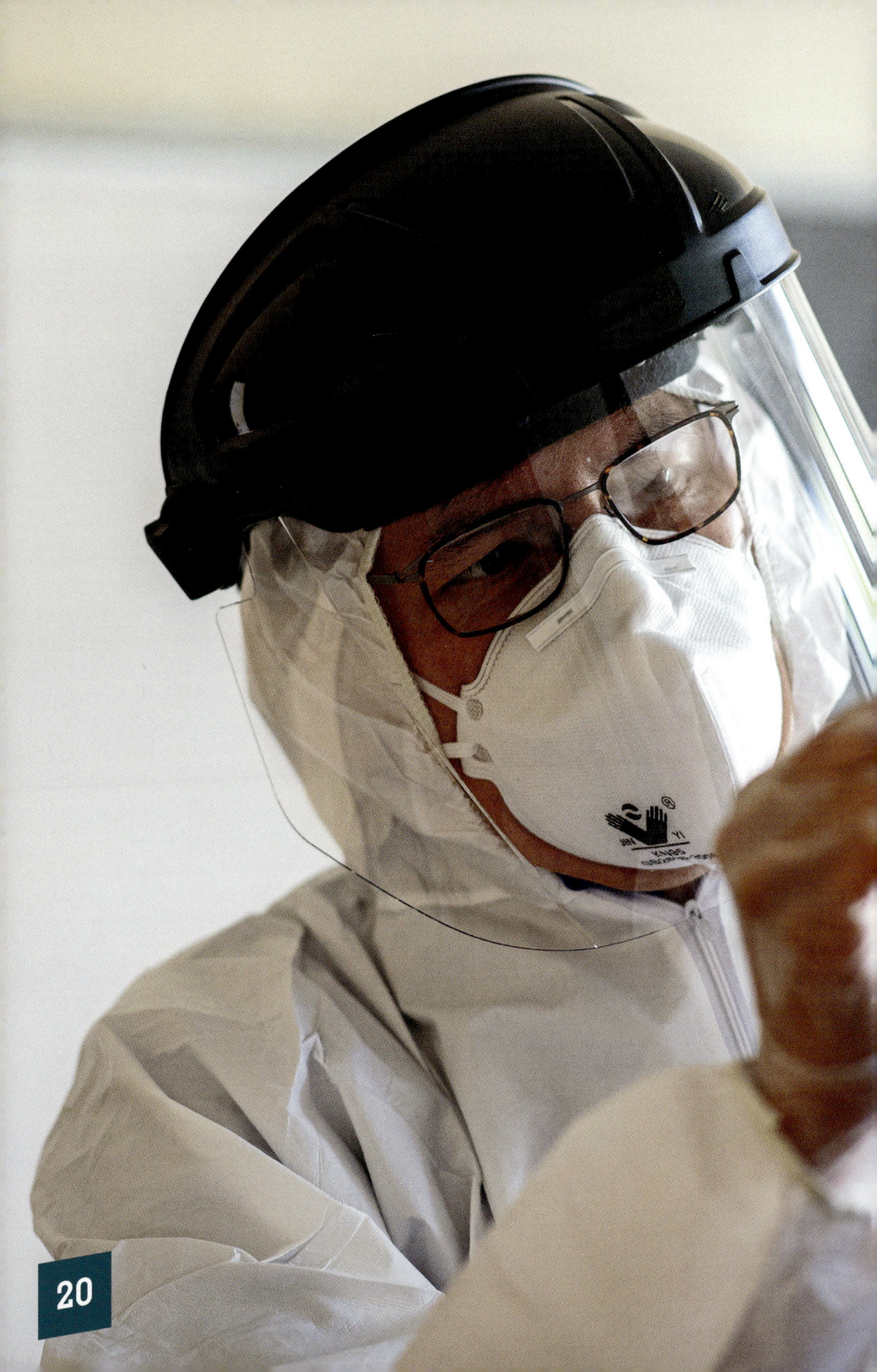

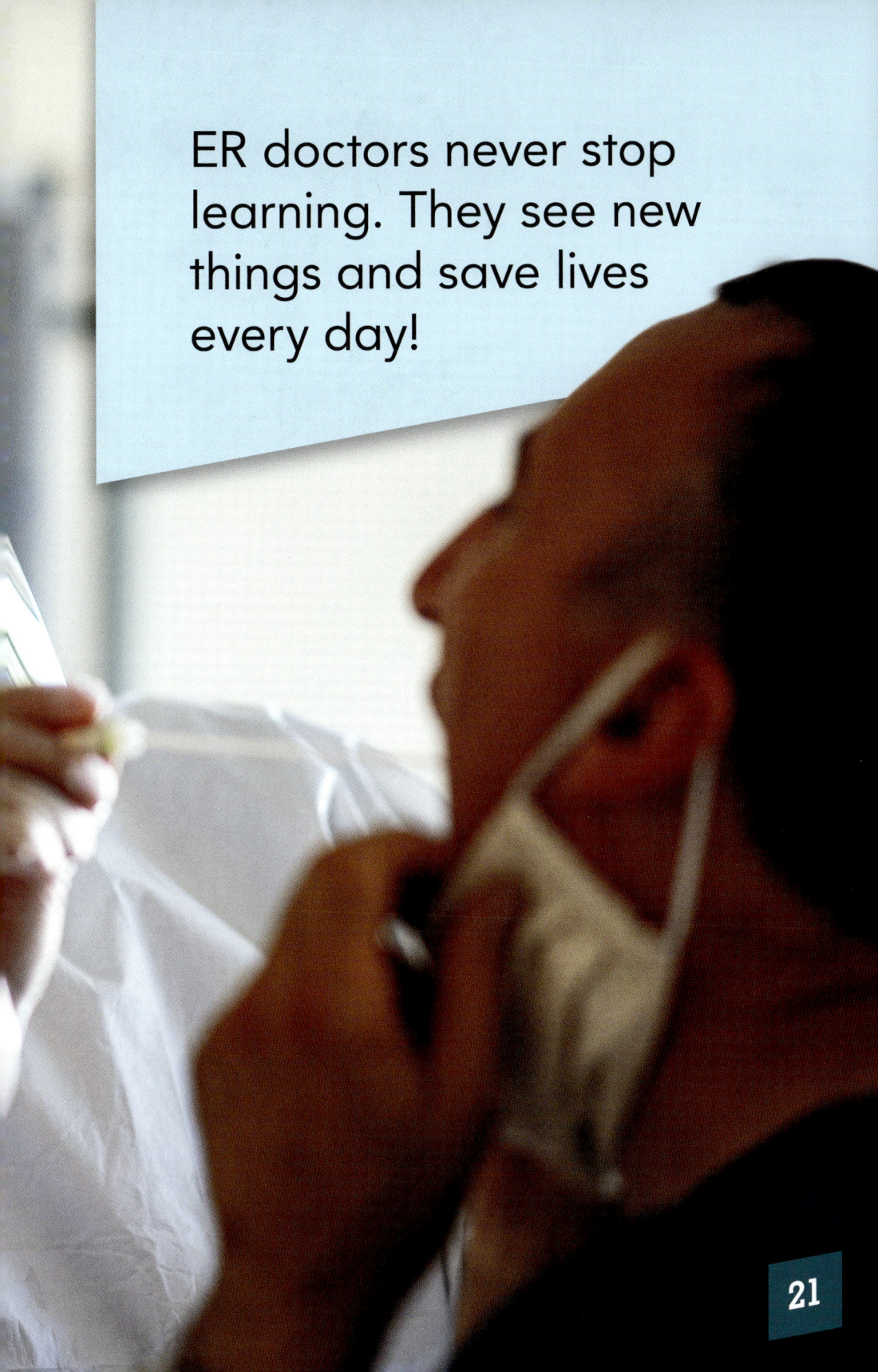

ER doctors never stop learning. They see new things and save lives every day!

More Facts

- ER doctors are also called emergency medicine specialists.

- There are more than 55,000 ER doctors in the US.

- About 140 million people visit an ER each year in the US.

Glossary

orthopedic – the branch of medicine dealing with the skeletal system and its associated muscles and joints.

refer – to send or direct to a source for help.

residency – a period of advanced medical training that normally follows graduation from medical school.

stabilize – to make stable.

victim – someone who is hurt or injured by a person or event.

Index

ailments 6, 14

duties 6, 11, 13, 14, 21

education 17, 18, 21

emergency room 5

medical school 17

patients 6, 11, 13, 14

referrals 14

surgery 13

Online Resources

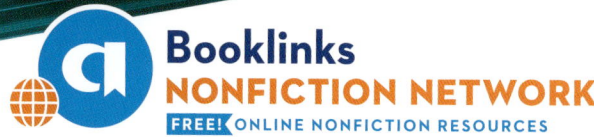

To learn more about ER doctors, please visit **abdobooklinks.com** or scan this QR code. These links are routinely monitored and updated to provide the most current information available.